NURSING

CARE

PLAN

WORKBOOK

NURSIAN COMMUNIT

CLIENT NAME _____

DATE INITIATED _____

ASSESSMENT

DIAGNOSIS

OUTCOMES

INTERVENTIONS

RATIONALE

EVALUATION

CLIENT NAME _____

DATE INITIATED _____

ASSESSMENT

DIAGNOSIS

OUTCOMES

INTERVENTIONS

RATIONALE

EVALUATION

CLIENT NAME _____

DATE INITIATED _____

ASSESSMENT

DIAGNOSIS

OUTCOMES

INTERVENTIONS

RATIONALE

EVALUATION

CLIENT NAME _____

DATE INITIATED _____

ASSESSMENT

DIAGNOSIS

OUTCOMES

INTERVENTIONS

RATIONALE

EVALUATION

CLIENT NAME _____

DATE INITIATED _____

ASSESSMENT

DIAGNOSIS

OUTCOMES

INTERVENTIONS

RATIONALE

EVALUATION

CLIENT NAME _____

DATE INITIATED _____

ASSESSMENT

DIAGNOSIS

OUTCOMES

INTERVENTIONS

RATIONALE

EVALUATION

CLIENT NAME _____

DATE INITIATED _____

ASSESSMENT

DIAGNOSIS

OUTCOMES

INTERVENTIONS

RATIONALE

EVALUATION

CLIENT NAME _____

DATE INITIATED _____

ASSESSMENT

DIAGNOSIS

OUTCOMES

CARE PLAN BY _____

INTERVENTIONS

RATIONALE

EVALUATION

CLIENT NAME _____

DATE INITIATED _____

ASSESSMENT

DIAGNOSIS

OUTCOMES

CARE PLAN BY

INTERVENTIONS

RATIONALE

EVALUATION

CLIENT NAME _____

DATE INITIATED _____

ASSESSMENT

DIAGNOSIS

OUTCOMES

INTERVENTIONS

RATIONALE

EVALUATION

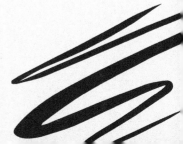

CLIENT NAME _____

DATE INITIATED _____

ASSESSMENT

DIAGNOSIS

OUTCOMES

INTERVENTIONS

RATIONALE

EVALUATION

CLIENT NAME _____

DATE INITIATED _____

ASSESSMENT

DIAGNOSIS

OUTCOMES

INTERVENTIONS

RATIONALE

EVALUATION

CLIENT NAME _____

DATE INITIATED _____

ASSESSMENT

DIAGNOSIS

OUTCOMES

INTERVENTIONS

RATIONALE

EVALUATION

CLIENT NAME _____

DATE INITIATED _____

ASSESSMENT

DIAGNOSIS

OUTCOMES

INTERVENTIONS

RATIONALE

EVALUATION

CLIENT NAME _____

DATE INITIATED _____

ASSESSMENT

DIAGNOSIS

OUTCOMES

INTERVENTIONS

RATIONALE

EVALUATION

CLIENT NAME _____

DATE INITIATED _____

ASSESSMENT

DIAGNOSIS

OUTCOMES

INTERVENTIONS

RATIONALE

EVALUATION

CLIENT NAME _____

DATE INITIATED _____

ASSESSMENT

DIAGNOSIS

OUTCOMES

INTERVENTIONS

RATIONALE

EVALUATION

CLIENT NAME _____

DATE INITIATED _____

ASSESSMENT

DIAGNOSIS

OUTCOMES

INTERVENTIONS

RATIONALE

EVALUATION

CLIENT NAME _____

DATE INITIATED _____

ASSESSMENT

DIAGNOSIS

OUTCOMES

CARE PLAN BY

INTERVENTIONS

RATIONALE

EVALUATION

CLIENT NAME _____

DATE INITIATED _____

ASSESSMENT

DIAGNOSIS

OUTCOMES

INTERVENTIONS

RATIONALE

EVALUATION

CLIENT NAME _____

DATE INITIATED _____

ASSESSMENT

DIAGNOSIS

OUTCOMES

CARE PLAN BY _____

INTERVENTIONS

RATIONALE

EVALUATION

CLIENT NAME _____

DATE INITIATED _____

ASSESSMENT

DIAGNOSIS

OUTCOMES

INTERVENTIONS

RATIONALE

EVALUATION

CLIENT NAME _____

DATE INITIATED _____

ASSESSMENT

DIAGNOSIS

OUTCOMES

INTERVENTIONS

RATIONALE

EVALUATION

CLIENT NAME _____

DATE INITIATED _____

ASSESSMENT

DIAGNOSIS

OUTCOMES

INTERVENTIONS

RATIONALE

EVALUATION

CLIENT NAME _____

DATE INITIATED _____

ASSESSMENT

DIAGNOSIS

OUTCOMES

INTERVENTIONS

RATIONALE

EVALUATION

CLIENT NAME _____

DATE INITIATED _____

ASSESSMENT

DIAGNOSIS

OUTCOMES

INTERVENTIONS

RATIONALE

EVALUATION

CLIENT NAME _____

DATE INITIATED _____

ASSESSMENT

DIAGNOSIS

OUTCOMES

RATIONALE

EVALUATION

CLIENT NAME _____

DATE INITIATED _____

ASSESSMENT

DIAGNOSIS

OUTCOMES

INTERVENTIONS

RATIONALE

EVALUATION

CLIENT NAME _____

DATE INITIATED _____

ASSESSMENT

DIAGNOSIS

OUTCOMES

INTERVENTIONS

RATIONALE

EVALUATION

CLIENT NAME _____

DATE INITIATED _____

ASSESSMENT

DIAGNOSIS

OUTCOMES

INTERVENTIONS

RATIONALE

EVALUATION

CLIENT NAME _____

DATE INITIATED _____

ASSESSMENT

DIAGNOSIS

OUTCOMES

INTERVENTIONS

RATIONALE

EVALUATION

CLIENT NAME _____

DATE INITIATED _____

ASSESSMENT

DIAGNOSIS

OUTCOMES

INTERVENTIONS

RATIONALE

EVALUATION

CLIENT NAME _____

DATE INITIATED _____

ASSESSMENT

DIAGNOSIS

OUTCOMES

INTERVENTIONS

RATIONALE

EVALUATION

CLIENT NAME _____

DATE INITIATED _____

ASSESSMENT

DIAGNOSIS

OUTCOMES

CARE PLAN BY

INTERVENTIONS

RATIONALE

EVALUATION

CLIENT NAME _____

DATE INITIATED _____

ASSESSMENT

DIAGNOSIS

OUTCOMES

INTERVENTIONS

RATIONALE

EVALUATION

CLIENT NAME _____

DATE INITIATED _____

ASSESSMENT

DIAGNOSIS

OUTCOMES

INTERVENTIONS

RATIONALE

EVALUATION

CLIENT NAME _____

DATE INITIATED _____

ASSESSMENT

DIAGNOSIS

OUTCOMES

INTERVENTIONS

RATIONALE

EVALUATION

CLIENT NAME _____

DATE INITIATED _____

ASSESSMENT

DIAGNOSIS

OUTCOMES

INTERVENTIONS

RATIONALE

EVALUATION

CLIENT NAME _____

DATE INITIATED _____

ASSESSMENT

DIAGNOSIS

OUTCOMES

CARE PLAN BY

INTERVENTIONS

RATIONALE

EVALUATION

CLIENT NAME _____

DATE INITIATED _____

ASSESSMENT

DIAGNOSIS

OUTCOMES

INTERVENTIONS

RATIONALE

EVALUATION

CLIENT NAME _____

DATE INITIATED _____

ASSESSMENT

DIAGNOSIS

OUTCOMES

RATIONALE

EVALUATION

CLIENT NAME _____

DATE INITIATED _____

ASSESSMENT

DIAGNOSIS

OUTCOMES

INTERVENTIONS

RATIONALE

EVALUATION

CLIENT NAME _____

DATE INITIATED _____

ASSESSMENT

DIAGNOSIS

OUTCOMES

CARE PLAN BY

INTERVENTIONS

RATIONALE

EVALUATION

CLIENT NAME _____

DATE INITIATED _____

ASSESSMENT

DIAGNOSIS

OUTCOMES

INTERVENTIONS

RATIONALE

EVALUATION

CLIENT NAME _____

DATE INITIATED _____

ASSESSMENT

DIAGNOSIS

OUTCOMES

INTERVENTIONS

RATIONALE

EVALUATION

CLIENT NAME _____

DATE INITIATED _____

ASSESSMENT

DIAGNOSIS

OUTCOMES

INTERVENTIONS

RATIONALE

EVALUATION

CLIENT NAME _____

DATE INITIATED _____

ASSESSMENT

DIAGNOSIS

OUTCOMES

INTERVENTIONS

RATIONALE

EVALUATION

CLIENT NAME _____

DATE INITIATED _____

ASSESSMENT

DIAGNOSIS

OUTCOMES

INTERVENTIONS

RATIONALE

EVALUATION

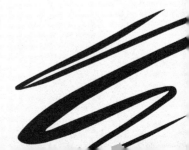

CLIENT NAME _____

DATE INITIATED _____

ASSESSMENT

DIAGNOSIS

OUTCOMES

INTERVENTIONS

RATIONALE

EVALUATION

CLIENT NAME _____

DATE INITIATED _____

ASSESSMENT

DIAGNOSIS

OUTCOMES

INTERVENTIONS

RATIONALE

EVALUATION

CLIENT NAME _____

DATE INITIATED _____

ASSESSMENT

DIAGNOSIS

OUTCOMES

INTERVENTIONS

RATIONALE

EVALUATION

CLIENT NAME _____

DATE INITIATED _____

ASSESSMENT

DIAGNOSIS

OUTCOMES

INTERVENTIONS

RATIONALE

EVALUATION

CLIENT NAME _____

DATE INITIATED _____

ASSESSMENT

DIAGNOSIS

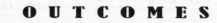

OUTCOMES

INTERVENTIONS

RATIONALE

EVALUATION

CLIENT NAME _____

DATE INITIATED _____

ASSESSMENT

DIAGNOSIS

OUTCOMES

INTERVENTIONS

RATIONALE

EVALUATION

CLIENT NAME _____

DATE INITIATED _____

ASSESSMENT

DIAGNOSIS

OUTCOMES

CARE PLAN BY

INTERVENTIONS

RATIONALE

EVALUATION

Made in the USA
Las Vegas, NV
15 April 2023